BE FIT IN 100 DAYS!

(FOOD JOURNAL)

Be fit in 100 days! (Food Journal)
Look and feel great while having in 100!
Primera Edición
© Mónica Carrasco, 2016

Manufactured in United States of America

ISBN–13: 978-1533190079

ISBN–10: 1533190070

BE FIT IN 100 DAYS!

(FOOD JOURNAL)

MÓNICA CARRASCO

LOOK AND FEEL GREAT WHILE HAVING FUN AND FITNESS IN 100 days!

FOREWORD

Have you ever been on a diet before? I have. My guess is you have at some point in your life and know, as I, it is not easy.

I am writing this to propose something that you can try that I guarantee will make you feel better and at the same time help you learn a lot about yourself! It is easy to follow and all you need is determination and will power to complete this 100 day program. It will not take too much of your time and at the end of the day the feeling of accomplishment will be incredible! Sooner or later you will be really happy and will be recommending it to your friends. I wish you the best because you deserve it!

ACKNOWLEDGEMENTS

I would like to thank my husband and my kids for being patient with me while I took many hours putting this journal together.

PURPOSE

The purpose of this program is to make you feel happy while you consume the food that you want as long as it is healthy to stay within your weight range. You should do this for positive health benefits and you will see that you will feel accomplished once it starts working for you. You will be able to reduce the amount of fat intake and this will reduce the risk of heart disease improving your lifestyle **(APPENDIX B).** You will learn to control yourself as far as the servings you need to consume, and you will also realize that the portions listed in the nutrition labels are the portions necessary to satisfy you. The problem comes in when we over eat and do not choose the right items. Well, I hope this will make a difference in your life because as an educator your SUCCESS IS MY HAPPINESS!!!

INTRODUCTION

I refer to it as the CALCULATOR REGIMEN. I call it like this because it is not really a "specific diet" or menu that you have to follow. Instead, it is YOU who decides what to eat (as long as it is healthy)!!! I have done it (successfully I would like to add) and truly believe it is a good way to get rid of extra weight. With the calculator regimen you are able to eat whatever you desire. You must, however, choose healthy natural foods and must not go over your allotted amount of grams per food group daily. All you need for this project is a calculator, a scale to weigh the food, and a scale to weigh yourself, my journal, and of course a well sharpened pencil ☺. Just make sure that when you weigh yourself you do it the same day of the week and at the same time.

When choosing the kind of food you desire to consume you must read the NUTRITION LABELS and look at the portions it recommends. You should stick to one portion or serving (depending on your calorie intake) and then record it in your journal. You will notice that some foods have too much of a particular compound. For example, almonds: I love almonds but they have way too many grams of fat per serving. One serving of almonds is 30 grams (approx. 24 almonds) and has 14 grams of FAT!!! It also has 6 grams of carbs and 6 grams of protein. In my opinion, the carbs and the proteins are ok but the fat is not. I only eat (on days I work out) 35 grams of fat. Eating one serving of almonds would put me at almost half of my allotted grams of fat in a day. This would not be a good choice. You must be wise in deciding what you eat.

In the first five days or so you will be able to determine how well (or not so well) you have been eating. But don't worry. It is okay to go over the amounts you need but remember to record it at the end of the day. By recording what you eat you will determine your daily eating pattern or routine. You will then be able to analyze your journal and decide what adjustments are necessary to achieve your goal. For example, if your goal is 150 grams/day of carbs and you went over, just adjust it for the next day.

HOW DOES IT WORK?

To get started you multiply by 13 (for women) times your desired weight (14 for men) to find out the daily amount of calories that you must consume to start. If you desire 200 pounds or over multiply by 11 or use a calorie calculator from the web.

One recommended is www.runnersworld.com/rybo. Thirteen and fourteen are numbers for people that are between lightly and moderately active. Now you will see how this program will really help you.

Example: (You are at 140 pounds and want to lose 10 pounds) 130 lbs X 13 = 1690 calories, the minimum and maximum amount you must eat daily. If you are exercising and you are burning 400 calories/day you are actually consuming 1,238 calories. As you lose weight, let's say you reach 130 lbs, you must multiply by 13 again and adjust your calories and grams again. This is actually how and the reason why you are losing weight and why this program works!

Eating right and exercising is the key to healthy life! In the journal section you will find a calculation sheet for this information and most importantly is to remember that less than 1200 calories for women and 1800 calories for men is not healthy and not recommended according to Health Experts.

EXAMPLE WORKSHEET FOR A WOMAN WHOSE DESIRED WEIGHT IS 130 POUNDS WITH SOME EXERCISE BURNING FROM 2000 TO 3500 CALS. PER WEEK.

CALORIES DISTRIBUTION: 50% CARBOHYDRATES, 30% PROTEINS, 20% FAT. (GOOD PLACE TO START)

STEP 1: TOTAL DAILY CALORIE INTAKE

MULTIPLY YOUR CURRENT WEIGHT BY 13:
EXAMPLE= 130 X 13 = **1,690 CALORIES/DAY**

STEP 2: DAILY GRAMS OF CARBOHYDRATES: 50%

50% OF THE TOTAL DAILY CALORIE INTAKE DIVIDED BY 4. (You will divide by 4 because it takes 4 calories to burn 1 gram of carbohydrate)
1,690 X 0.50 = **845 CALORIES**
845 DIVIDED BY 4 = **211 GRAMS**

STEP 3: DAILY GRAMS OF FAT: 20%

20% OF THE TOTAL DAILY CALORIE INTAKE DIVIDED BY 9. (You will divide by 9 because it takes 9 calories to burn 1 gram of fat)
1,690 X 0.20 = **338 CALORIES**
338 DIVIDED BY 9 = **38 GRAMS**

STEP 4: DAILY GRAMS OF PROTEIN: 30%

30% OF THE TOTAL DAILY CALORIE INTAKE DIVIDED BY 4. (You will divide by 4 because it takes 4 calories to burn 1 gram of protein)
1,690 X 0.30 = **507 CALORIES**
507 DIVIDED BY 4 = **127 GRAMS**

WHY DO YOU HAVE TO DIVIDE BY 4 OR 9?

It's because it takes 4 calories of carbohydrates to burn one gram of carbohydrates. The same situation applies to proteins. In the case of fat, more calories are needed. It takes 9 calories of fat to burn one gram of it. This is the reason why fat deposits for a long time in our bodies and it requires more energy to burn it.

LET'S GET STARTED!

The first thing you must do is to learn how to use the NUTRITION FACTS labels in food items.

This is an easy task to do since you must only copy the following information:

Number of calories –number of fat in grams– number of carbohydrates in grams –number of proteins in grams– number of fiber in grams –the milligrams of sodium– milligrams of cholesterol and the food description.

These are the numbers you must record in your journal and add them up to reach your desired calories/grams intake. If the portion says ½ cup or ¼ of a cup, you must be attentive because if you eat two portions you must multiply everything by two. Following is an example of a Nutrition Label Fact. Please read it very carefully and make sure you understand.

Serving Size &
Calories

Limit These
Nutrients

Get Enough
of These

Daily Value
Recommendations

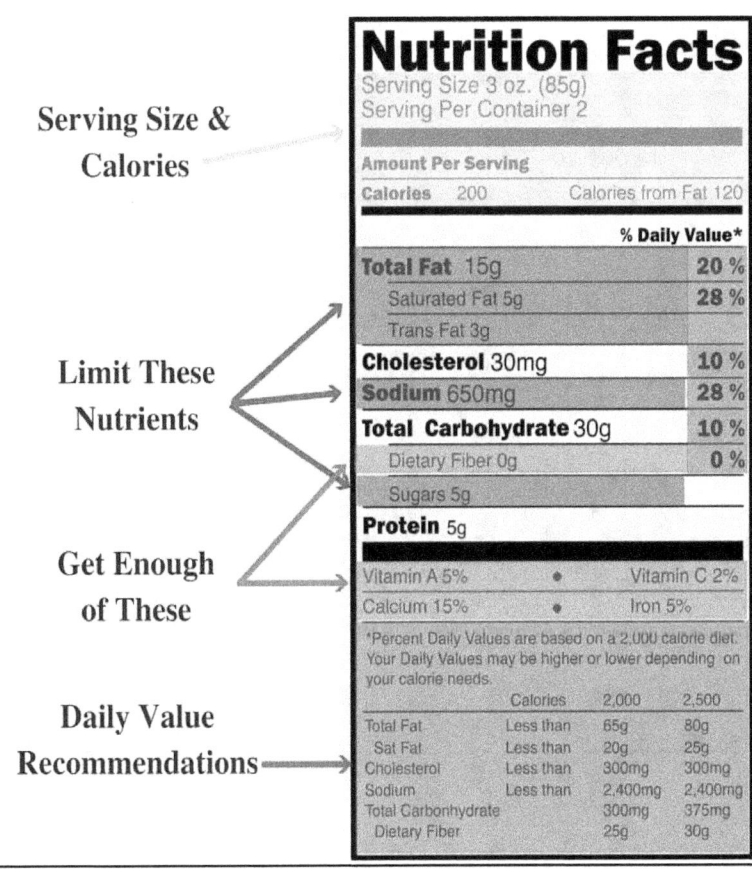

Nutrition Facts
Serving Size 3 oz. (85g)
Serving Per Container 2

Amount Per Serving

Calories 200   Calories from Fat 120

% Daily Value*

Total Fat 15g	**20 %**
Saturated Fat 5g	**28 %**
Trans Fat 3g	
Cholesterol 30mg	**10 %**
Sodium 650mg	**28 %**
Total Carbohydrate 30g	**10 %**
Dietary Fiber 0g	**0 %**
Sugars 5g	

Protein 5g

Vitamin A 5%   •   Vitamin C 2%

Calcium 15%   •   Iron 5%

*Percent Daily Values are based on a 2,000 calorie diet.
Your Daily Values may be higher or lower depending on
your calorie needs.

	Calories	2,000	2,500
Total Fat	Less than	65g	80g
Sat Fat	Less than	20g	25g
Cholesterol	Less than	300mg	300mg
Sodium	Less than	2,400mg	2,400mg
Total Carbohydrate		300mg	375mg
Dietary Fiber		25g	30g

These are the steps to follow in recording your information:

STEP 1: Record today's date, day and your present weight.

STEP 2: Record your goals for that day.

EXAMPLE

DAILY	Calories	Fat (g)	Carbs (g)	Fiber (g)	Protein (g)	Sodium (mg)	Cholesterol (mg)
GOAL	1690cals	38g	130g	25g-38g	38g	1500-2400mg	300mg

STEP 3: Record what you really consume that day.

FOOD DESCRIPTION	2 scoops of protein shake	1 slice of Bread	2 Tbsp Peanut butter
CALORIES	260	80	190
CARBS(g)	3	15	8
PROTEIN(g)	54	4	7
FAT	1.5	1	16
FIBER	0	1	2
SODIUM	150	115	135
CHOLESTEROL	40	0	0

STEP 4: Record the amount water consumed. For men is 3 liters (13 cups) of total beverages/day and for women is 2.2 liters (9 cups) of total beverages per day.

STEP 5: Make an analysis and compare it to your goal. Repeat for 100 days or more!

You will determine in the first few days where you stand with the serving you consume daily. As days go by you will become better at measuring the amounts and portions you need. If you feel you deserve a day off, take it! You'll see that you will still take pounds off because what you are doing is creating a deficit of calories and this is what is really helping you shed your extra pounds. It is perfectly fine to lose from ¼ pound to 2 pounds of body fat per week depending on how many calories you burnt exercising that week (3500 cals/1 pound of fat). Don't go crazy trying to lose weight too fast because it is not healthy. Besides, this is a healthier lifestyle that you are acquiring. One hundred days is more than enough for you to memorize the way you must eat. The purpose of this journal is to write and imprint in your mind the portions you should eat. If you need more than one hundred days it's okay too. Just use another journal. This will teach you to control your portions which is where the secret lies.

RECORDING YOUR INFORMATION

Make sure you record all the numbers accordingly. In you journal you will see rows for the following:

FOOD, CALORIES, CARBS, FIBER, PROTEIN, SODIUM, CHOLESTEROL AND FAT **(APPENDIX G, sample log).**

Fiber is very important in our diet because we do not digest it. It goes right through our digestive system bonding and taking with it fat molecules. Record your sodium and cholesterol as well. Sodium is an important electrolyte and mineral that helps maintain balance inside and out of the cells including nerve and muscle cells. Limit your daily sodium intake to 1500mg minimum and a maximum of 2400mg. Government guidelines recommends to intake less than 300mg per day of cholesterol.

STAY AWAY!!!

It's important to consume very low amounts of saturated fats (less than 7% of daily calories recommended by the American Heart Association, **AHA**), trans-fat, white carbohydrates, processed foods and refined sugars.

MUST DO!

- Take a multivitamin daily. Please consult with your general doctor first.
  (APPENDIX D AND E)
- Measure your food.
- Weigh yourself once a week at the same time.
- Purchase items with a nutritional label.
- Eat at least 25g for women and 38 grams for men of fiber on a daily basis. (pick whole grain vs. white starch food)
- Exercise and burn from 200 to 1000 calories at least 3 times/week.
  3500 calories burnt represent one pound of body fat lost/ week.
- Choose plenty of vegetables and whole grain products. (APPENDIX F)
- Consume moderate amount of fresh fruit daily. The USDA recommends two cups per day. (APPENDIX F)
- Consume plenty amount of water. The Institute of Medicine determined that an adequate intake of water for men is roughly about 13 cups (3 liters) of total beverages a day and for women is about 9 cups (2.2 liters) of total beverages a day.

NUTRIENT BREAKDOWN WORKSHEET
WOMAN (13) MAN (14). 50%-30%-20%.
OPTIONAL PERCENTAGES
(you can change these percentages)

STEP 1: TOTAL DAILY CALORIE INTAKE
MULTIPLY YOUR DESIRED WEIGHT BY 13:

_____ X 13/14 =   CALORIES INTAKE/DAY

STEP 2: DAILY GRAMS OF CARBOHYDRATES: 50% OF THE TOTAL DAILY CALORIE INTAKE DIVIDED BY 4.

_____ X 0.50 =   CALORIES OF CARBS.
_____ DIVIDED BY 4 (4 calories to burn 1 gram of carbs) = GRAMS OF CARBS.

STEP 3: DAILY GRAMS OF FAT: 20%
20% OF THE TOTAL DAILY CALORIE INTAKE DIVIDED BY 9.

_____ X 0.20 =   CALORIES OF FAT. _____
DIVIDED BY 9 (9 calories to burn 1 gram of fat) =   GRAMS OF FAT.

STEP 4: DAILY GRAMS OF PROTEIN: 30%
30% OF THE TOTAL DAILY CALORIE INTAKE DIVIDED BY 4.

_____ X 0.30 =   CALORIES OF PROTEIN.
_____ DIVIDED BY 4 (4 calories to burn 1 gram of protein) = GRAMS OF PROTEIN.

PROTEIN (GRAMS) _____ g
FAT (GRAMS) _____ g
CARBOHYDRATES (GRAMS) _____ g

NUTRIENT BREAKDOWN WORKSHEET
WOMAN (13) MAN (14). 50%-30%-20%.
OPTIONAL PERCENTAGES
(you can change these percentages)

STEP 1: TOTAL DAILY CALORIE INTAKE
MULTIPLY YOUR DESIRED WEIGHT BY 13:

_____ X 13/14 =   CALORIES INTAKE/DAY

STEP 2: DAILY GRAMS OF CARBOHYDRATES: 50% OF THE
TOTAL DAILY CALORIE INTAKE DIVIDED BY 4.

_____ X 0.50 =   CALORIES OF CARBS.
_____DIVIDED BY 4 (4 calories to burn 1 gram of carbs) =
GRAMS OF CARBS.

STEP 3: DAILY GRAMS OF FAT: 20%
20% OF THE TOTAL DAILY CALORIE INTAKE DIVIDED BY
9.

_____X 0.20 =   CALORIES OF FAT. _____
DIVIDED BY 9 (9 calories to burn 1 gram of fat) =   GRAMS
OF FAT.

STEP 4: DAILY GRAMS OF PROTEIN: 30%
30% OF THE TOTAL DAILY CALORIE INTAKE DIVIDED BY
4.

_____ X 0.30 =   CALORIES OF PROTEIN.
_____DIVIDED BY 4 (4 calories to burn 1 gram of protein) =
GRAMS OF PROTEIN.

PROTEIN (GRAMS) _____g
FAT (GRAMS) _____g
CARBOHYDRATES (GRAMS)_____g

NUTRIENT BREAKDOWN WORKSHEET
WOMAN (13) MAN (14). 50%-30%-20%.
OPTIONAL PERCENTAGES
(you can change these percentages)

STEP 1: TOTAL DAILY CALORIE INTAKE
MULTIPLY YOUR DESIRED WEIGHT BY 13:

_____ X 13/14 =   CALORIES INTAKE/DAY

STEP 2: DAILY GRAMS OF CARBOHYDRATES: 50% OF THE
TOTAL DAILY CALORIE INTAKE DIVIDED BY 4.

_____ X 0.50 =   CALORIES OF CARBS.
_____DIVIDED BY 4 (4 calories to burn 1 gram of carbs) =
GRAMS OF CARBS.

STEP 3: DAILY GRAMS OF FAT: 20%
20% OF THE TOTAL DAILY CALORIE INTAKE DIVIDED BY
9.

_____X 0.20 =   CALORIES OF FAT. _____
DIVIDED BY 9 (9 calories to burn 1 gram of fat) =   GRAMS
OF FAT.

STEP 4: DAILY GRAMS OF PROTEIN: 30%
30% OF THE TOTAL DAILY CALORIE INTAKE DIVIDED BY
4.

_____ X 0.30 =   CALORIES OF PROTEIN.
_____DIVIDED BY 4 (4 calories to burn 1 gram of protein) =
GRAMS OF PROTEIN.

PROTEIN (GRAMS) _____g
FAT (GRAMS) _____g
CARBOHYDRATES (GRAMS)_____g

NUTRIENT BREAKDOWN WORKSHEET
WOMAN (13) MAN (14). 50%-30%-20%.
OPTIONAL PERCENTAGES
(you can change these percentages)

STEP 1: TOTAL DAILY CALORIE INTAKE
MULTIPLY YOUR DESIRED WEIGHT BY 13:

_____ X 13/14 =   CALORIES INTAKE/DAY

STEP 2: DAILY GRAMS OF CARBOHYDRATES: 50% OF THE
TOTAL DAILY CALORIE INTAKE DIVIDED BY 4.

_____ X 0.50 =   CALORIES OF CARBS.
_____DIVIDED BY 4 (4 calories to burn 1 gram of carbs) =
GRAMS OF CARBS.

STEP 3: DAILY GRAMS OF FAT: 20%
20% OF THE TOTAL DAILY CALORIE INTAKE DIVIDED BY
9.

_____X 0.20 =   CALORIES OF FAT. _____
DIVIDED BY 9 (9 calories to burn 1 gram of fat) =   GRAMS
OF FAT.

STEP 4: DAILY GRAMS OF PROTEIN: 30%
30% OF THE TOTAL DAILY CALORIE INTAKE DIVIDED BY
4.

_____ X 0.30 =   CALORIES OF PROTEIN.
_____DIVIDED BY 4 (4 calories to burn 1 gram of protein) =
GRAMS OF PROTEIN.

PROTEIN (GRAMS) _____g
FAT (GRAMS) _____g
CARBOHYDRATES (GRAMS)_____g

NUTRIENT BREAKDOWN WORKSHEET
WOMAN (13) MAN (14). 50%-30%-20%.
OPTIONAL PERCENTAGES
(you can change these percentages)

STEP 1: TOTAL DAILY CALORIE INTAKE
MULTIPLY YOUR DESIRED WEIGHT BY 13:

_____ X 13/14 =   CALORIES INTAKE/DAY

STEP 2: DAILY GRAMS OF CARBOHYDRATES: 50% OF THE
TOTAL DAILY CALORIE INTAKE DIVIDED BY 4.

_____ X 0.50 =   CALORIES OF CARBS.
_____DIVIDED BY 4 (4 calories to burn 1 gram of carbs) =
GRAMS OF CARBS.

STEP 3: DAILY GRAMS OF FAT: 20%
20% OF THE TOTAL DAILY CALORIE INTAKE DIVIDED BY
9.

_____X 0.20 =   CALORIES OF FAT. _____
DIVIDED BY 9 (9 calories to burn 1 gram of fat) =   GRAMS
OF FAT.

STEP 4: DAILY GRAMS OF PROTEIN: 30%
30% OF THE TOTAL DAILY CALORIE INTAKE DIVIDED BY
4.

_____ X 0.30 =   CALORIES OF PROTEIN.
_____DIVIDED BY 4 (4 calories to burn 1 gram of protein) =
GRAMS OF PROTEIN.

PROTEIN (GRAMS) _____g
FAT (GRAMS) _____g
CARBOHYDRATES (GRAMS)_____g

NUTRIENT BREAKDOWN WORKSHEET
WOMAN (13) MAN (14). 50%-30%-20%.
OPTIONAL PERCENTAGES
(you can change these percentages)

STEP 1: TOTAL DAILY CALORIE INTAKE
MULTIPLY YOUR DESIRED WEIGHT BY 13:

_____ X 13/14 =   CALORIES INTAKE/DAY

STEP 2: DAILY GRAMS OF CARBOHYDRATES: 50% OF THE
TOTAL DAILY CALORIE INTAKE DIVIDED BY 4.

_____ X 0.50 =   CALORIES OF CARBS.
_____DIVIDED BY 4 (4 calories to burn 1 gram of carbs) =
GRAMS OF CARBS.

STEP 3: DAILY GRAMS OF FAT: 20%
20% OF THE TOTAL DAILY CALORIE INTAKE DIVIDED BY
9.

_____X 0.20 =   CALORIES OF FAT. _____
DIVIDED BY 9 (9 calories to burn 1 gram of fat) =   GRAMS
OF FAT.

STEP 4: DAILY GRAMS OF PROTEIN: 30%
30% OF THE TOTAL DAILY CALORIE INTAKE DIVIDED BY
4.

_____ X 0.30 =   CALORIES OF PROTEIN.
_____DIVIDED BY 4 (4 calories to burn 1 gram of protein) =
GRAMS OF PROTEIN.

PROTEIN (GRAMS) _____g
FAT (GRAMS) _____g
CARBOHYDRATES (GRAMS)_____g

NUTRIENT BREAKDOWN WORKSHEET
WOMAN (13) MAN (14). 50%-30%-20%.
OPTIONAL PERCENTAGES
(you can change these percentages)

STEP 1: TOTAL DAILY CALORIE INTAKE
MULTIPLY YOUR DESIRED WEIGHT BY 13:

_____ X 13/14 =   CALORIES INTAKE/DAY

STEP 2: DAILY GRAMS OF CARBOHYDRATES: 50% OF THE
TOTAL DAILY CALORIE INTAKE DIVIDED BY 4.

_____ X 0.50 =   CALORIES OF CARBS.
_____DIVIDED BY 4 (4 calories to burn 1 gram of carbs) =
GRAMS OF CARBS.

STEP 3: DAILY GRAMS OF FAT: 20%
20% OF THE TOTAL DAILY CALORIE INTAKE DIVIDED BY
9.

_____X 0.20 =   CALORIES OF FAT. _____
DIVIDED BY 9 (9 calories to burn 1 gram of fat) =   GRAMS
OF FAT.

STEP 4: DAILY GRAMS OF PROTEIN: 30%
30% OF THE TOTAL DAILY CALORIE INTAKE DIVIDED BY
4.

_____ X 0.30 =   CALORIES OF PROTEIN.
_____DIVIDED BY 4 (4 calories to burn 1 gram of protein) =
GRAMS OF PROTEIN.

PROTEIN (GRAMS) _____g
FAT (GRAMS) _____g
CARBOHYDRATES (GRAMS)_____g

NUTRIENT BREAKDOWN WORKSHEET
WOMAN (13) MAN (14). 50%-30%-20%.
OPTIONAL PERCENTAGES
(you can change these percentages)

STEP 1: TOTAL DAILY CALORIE INTAKE
MULTIPLY YOUR DESIRED WEIGHT BY 13:

_____ X 13/14 =   CALORIES INTAKE/DAY

STEP 2: DAILY GRAMS OF CARBOHYDRATES: 50% OF THE
TOTAL DAILY CALORIE INTAKE DIVIDED BY 4.

_____ X 0.50 =   CALORIES OF CARBS.
_____DIVIDED BY 4 (4 calories to burn 1 gram of carbs) =
GRAMS OF CARBS.

STEP 3: DAILY GRAMS OF FAT: 20%
20% OF THE TOTAL DAILY CALORIE INTAKE DIVIDED BY
9.

_____X 0.20 =   CALORIES OF FAT. _____
DIVIDED BY 9 (9 calories to burn 1 gram of fat) =   GRAMS
OF FAT.

STEP 4: DAILY GRAMS OF PROTEIN: 30%
30% OF THE TOTAL DAILY CALORIE INTAKE DIVIDED BY
4.

_____ X 0.30 =   CALORIES OF PROTEIN.
_____DIVIDED BY 4 (4 calories to burn 1 gram of protein) =
GRAMS OF PROTEIN.

PROTEIN (GRAMS) _____g
FAT (GRAMS) _____g
CARBOHYDRATES (GRAMS)_____g

NUTRIENT BREAKDOWN WORKSHEET
WOMAN (13) MAN (14). 50%-30%-20%.
OPTIONAL PERCENTAGES
(you can change these percentages)

STEP 1: TOTAL DAILY CALORIE INTAKE
MULTIPLY YOUR DESIRED WEIGHT BY 13:

_____ X 13/14 =   CALORIES INTAKE/DAY

STEP 2: DAILY GRAMS OF CARBOHYDRATES: 50% OF THE
TOTAL DAILY CALORIE INTAKE DIVIDED BY 4.

_____ X 0.50 =   CALORIES OF CARBS.
_____DIVIDED BY 4 (4 calories to burn 1 gram of carbs) =
GRAMS OF CARBS.

STEP 3: DAILY GRAMS OF FAT: 20%
20% OF THE TOTAL DAILY CALORIE INTAKE DIVIDED BY
9.

_____X 0.20 =   CALORIES OF FAT. _____
DIVIDED BY 9 (9 calories to burn 1 gram of fat) =   GRAMS
OF FAT.

STEP 4: DAILY GRAMS OF PROTEIN: 30%
30% OF THE TOTAL DAILY CALORIE INTAKE DIVIDED BY
4.

_____ X 0.30 =   CALORIES OF PROTEIN.
_____DIVIDED BY 4 (4 calories to burn 1 gram of protein) =
GRAMS OF PROTEIN.

PROTEIN (GRAMS) _____g
FAT (GRAMS) _____g
CARBOHYDRATES (GRAMS)_____g

NUTRIENT BREAKDOWN WORKSHEET
WOMAN (13) MAN (14). 50%-30%-20%.
OPTIONAL PERCENTAGES
(you can change these percentages)

STEP 1: TOTAL DAILY CALORIE INTAKE
MULTIPLY YOUR DESIRED WEIGHT BY 13:

_____ X 13/14 =   CALORIES INTAKE/DAY

STEP 2: DAILY GRAMS OF CARBOHYDRATES: 50% OF THE
TOTAL DAILY CALORIE INTAKE DIVIDED BY 4.

_____ X 0.50 =   CALORIES OF CARBS.
_____DIVIDED BY 4 (4 calories to burn 1 gram of carbs) =
GRAMS OF CARBS.

STEP 3: DAILY GRAMS OF FAT: 20%
20% OF THE TOTAL DAILY CALORIE INTAKE DIVIDED BY
9.

_____X 0.20 =   CALORIES OF FAT. _____
DIVIDED BY 9 (9 calories to burn 1 gram of fat) =   GRAMS
OF FAT.

STEP 4: DAILY GRAMS OF PROTEIN: 30%
30% OF THE TOTAL DAILY CALORIE INTAKE DIVIDED BY
4.

_____ X 0.30 =   CALORIES OF PROTEIN.
_____DIVIDED BY 4 (4 calories to burn 1 gram of protein) =
GRAMS OF PROTEIN.

PROTEIN (GRAMS) _____g
FAT (GRAMS) _____g
CARBOHYDRATES (GRAMS)_____g

KEY WORDS

Cals = Calories

Carbs = Carbohydrates

Fib = Fiber

Prot = Protein

Fat = Fat

Sod = Sodium

Chol = Cholesterol

Day # | Date:
Weight:
Time:
Water (oz):

Food description	Cals	F a t	C a r b s	F i b	P r o t	S o d	Ch o l
		(g)	(g)	(g)	(g)	(mg)	(mg)
Breakfast							
Snack							
Lunch							
Snack							
Dinner							
Total Calories Consumed							

Daily Physical Activity_____

Daily Calories burned_____

Formula: (Calories consumed — Calories burned) =
Total calories intake per day

_____ = _____

Day #   Date:
Weight:
Time:
Water (oz):

Food description	Cals	Fat (g)	Carbs (g)	Fib (g)	Prot (g)	Sod (mg)	Chol (mg)
Breakfast							
Snack							
Lunch							
Snack							
Dinner							
Total Calories Consumed							

Daily Physical Activity_____

Daily Calories burned_____

Formula: (Calories consumed — Calories burned) =
Total calories intake per day

_____ = _____

Day #	Date:
	Weight:
	Time:
	Water (oz):

Food description	Cals	F a t	C a r b s	F i b	P r o t	S o d	Ch o l
		(g)	(g)	(g)	(g)	(mg)	(mg)
Breakfast							
Snack							
Lunch							
Snack							
Dinner							
Total Calories Consumed							

Daily Physical Activity_____

Daily Calories burned_____

**Formula: (Calories consumed — Calories burned) =
Total calories intake per day**

_____ = _____

Day # | Date:
Weight:
Time:
Water (oz):

Food description	Cals	Fat	Carbs	Fib	Prot	Sod	Chol
		(g)	(g)	(g)	(g)	(mg)	(mg)
Breakfast							
Snack							
Lunch							
Snack							
Dinner							
Total Calories Consumed							

Daily Physical Activity_____

Daily Calories burned_____

Formula: (Calories consumed — Calories burned) =
Total calories intake per day

_____ = _____

Day # | Date:
Weight:
Time:
Water (oz):

Food description	Cals	Fat	Carbs	Fib	Prot	Sod	Chol
		(g)	(g)	(g)	(g)	(mg)	(mg)
Breakfast							
Snack							
Lunch							
Snack							
Dinner							
Total Calories Consumed							

Daily Physical Activity_____

Daily Calories burned_____

Formula: (Calories consumed — Calories burned) =
Total calories intake per day

_____ = _____

Day #	Date: Weight: Time: Water (oz):

Food description	Cals	F a t	C a r b s	F i b	P r o t	S o d	Ch o l
		(g)	(g)	(g)	(g)	(mg)	(mg)
Breakfast							
Snack							
Lunch							
Snack							
Dinner							
Total Calories Consumed							

Daily Physical Activity_____

Daily Calories burned_____

Formula: (Calories consumed — Calories burned) =
Total calories intake per day

_____ = _____

Day
#

Date:
Weight:
Time:
Water (oz):

Food description	Cals	F a t (g)	C a r b s (g)	F i b (g)	P r o t (g)	S o d (mg)	Ch o l (mg)
Breakfast							
Snack							
Lunch							
Snack							
Dinner							
Total Calories Consumed							

Daily Physical Activity_____

Daily Calories burned_____

Formula: (Calories consumed — Calories burned) =
Total calories intake per day

_____ = _____

Day # | Date:
Weight:
Time:
Water (oz):

Food description	Cals	F a t	C a r b s	F i b	P r o t	S o d	Ch o l
		(g)	(g)	(g)	(g)	(mg)	(mg)
Breakfast							
Snack							
Lunch							
Snack							
Dinner							
Total Calories Consumed							

Daily Physical Activity_____

Daily Calories burned_____

Formula: (Calories consumed — Calories burned) =
Total calories intake per day

_____ = _____

Day #	Date: Weight: Time: Water (oz):

Food description	Cals	F a t	C a r b s	F i b	P r o t	S o d	Ch o l
		(g)	(g)	(g)	(g)	(mg)	(mg)
Breakfast							
Snack							
Lunch							
Snack							
Dinner							
Total Calories Consumed							

Daily Physical Activity_____

Daily Calories burned_____

Formula: (Calories consumed — Calories burned) =
Total calories intake per day

_____ = _____

Day #

Date:
Weight:
Time:
Water (oz):

Food description	Cals	Fat	Carbs	Fib	Prot	Sod	Chol
		(g)	(g)	(g)	(g)	(mg)	(mg)
Breakfast							
Snack							
Lunch							
Snack							
Dinner							
Total Calories Consumed							

Daily Physical Activity_____

Daily Calories burned_____

Formula: (Calories consumed — Calories burned) =
Total calories intake per day

_____ = _____

Day #	Date: Weight: Time: Water (oz):

Food description	Cals	F a t	C a r b s	F i b	P r o t	S o d	Ch o l
		(g)	(g)	(g)	(g)	(mg)	(mg)
Breakfast							
Snack							
Lunch							
Snack							
Dinner							
Total Calories Consumed							

Daily Physical Activity_____

Daily Calories burned_____

Formula: (Calories consumed − Calories burned) =
Total calories intake per day

_____ = _____

Day #   Date:
         Weight:
         Time:
         Water (oz):

Food description	Cals	Fat	Carbs	Fib	Prot	Sod	Chol
		(g)	(g)	(g)	(g)	(mg)	(mg)
Breakfast							
Snack							
Lunch							
Snack							
Dinner							
Total Calories Consumed							

Daily Physical Activity_____

Daily Calories burned_____

Formula: (Calories consumed — Calories burned) =
Total calories intake per day

_____ = _____

Day # Date:
Weight:
Time:
Water (oz):

Food description	Cals	Fat	Carbs	Fib	Prot	Sod	Chol
		(g)	(g)	(g)	(g)	(mg)	(mg)
Breakfast							
Snack							
Lunch							
Snack							
Dinner							
Total Calories Consumed							

Daily Physical Activity_____

Daily Calories burned_____

**Formula: (Calories consumed — Calories burned) =
Total calories intake per day**

_____ = _____

Day # | Date:
Weight:
Time:
Water (oz):

Food description	Cals	Fat (g)	Carbs (g)	Fib (g)	Prot (g)	Sod (mg)	Chol (mg)
Breakfast							
Snack							
Lunch							
Snack							
Dinner							
Total Calories Consumed							

Daily Physical Activity_____

Daily Calories burned_____

Formula: (Calories consumed — Calories burned) =
Total calories intake per day

_____ = _____

Day # | Date:
Weight:
Time:
Water (oz):

Food description	Cals	F a t (g)	C a r b s (g)	F i b (g)	P r o t (g)	S o d (mg)	Ch o l (mg)
Breakfast							
Snack							
Lunch							
Snack							
Dinner							
Total Calories Consumed							

Daily Physical Activity_____

Daily Calories burned_____

Formula: (Calories consumed — Calories burned) =
Total calories intake per day

_____ = _____

Day #

Date:
Weight:
Time:
Water (oz):

Food description	Cals	Fat	Carbs	Fib	Prot	Sod	Chol
		(g)	(g)	(g)	(g)	(mg)	(mg)
Breakfast							
Snack							
Lunch							
Snack							
Dinner							
Total Calories Consumed							

Daily Physical Activity_____

Daily Calories burned_____

Formula: (Calories consumed — Calories burned) =
Total calories intake per day

_____ = _____

Day # | Date:
Weight:
Time:
Water (oz):

Food description	Cals	F a t	C a r b s	F i b	P r o t	S o d	Ch o l
		(g)	(g)	(g)	(g)	(mg)	(mg)
Breakfast							
Snack							
Lunch							
Snack							
Dinner							
Total Calories Consumed							

Daily Physical Activity_____

Daily Calories burned_____

Formula: (Calories consumed — Calories burned) =
Total calories intake per day

_____ = _____

Day # Date:
Weight:
Time:
Water (oz):

Food description	Cals	Fat	Carbs	Fib	Prot	Sod	Chol
		(g)	(g)	(g)	(g)	(mg)	(mg)
Breakfast							
Snack							
Lunch							
Snack							
Dinner							
Total Calories Consumed							

Daily Physical Activity_____

Daily Calories burned_____

Formula: (Calories consumed — Calories burned) =
Total calories intake per day

_____ = _____

Day #

Date:
Weight:
Time:
Water (oz):

Food description	Cals	F a t (g)	C a r b s (g)	F i b (g)	P r o t (g)	S o d (mg)	Ch o l (mg)
Breakfast							
Snack							
Lunch							
Snack							
Dinner							
Total Calories Consumed							

Daily Physical Activity_____

Daily Calories burned_____

Formula: (Calories consumed — Calories burned) =
Total calories intake per day

_____ = _____

Day #   Date:
         Weight:
         Time:
         Water (oz):

Food description	Cals	Fat	Carbs	Fib	Prot	Sod	Chol
		(g)	(g)	(g)	(g)	(mg)	(mg)
Breakfast							
Snack							
Lunch							
Snack							
Dinner							
Total Calories Consumed							

Daily Physical Activity_____

Daily Calories burned_____

Formula: (Calories consumed — Calories burned) =
Total calories intake per day

_____ = _____

Day #	Date: Weight: Time: Water (oz):

Food description	Cals	F a t (g)	C a r b s (g)	F i b (g)	P r o t (g)	S o d (mg)	Ch o l (mg)
Breakfast							
Snack							
Lunch							
Snack							
Dinner							
Total Calories Consumed							

Daily Physical Activity_____

Daily Calories burned_____

Formula: (Calories consumed — Calories burned) =
Total calories intake per day

_____ = _____

Day # Date:
Weight:
Time:
Water (oz):

Food description	Cals	Fat	Carbs	Fib	Prot	Sod	Chol
		(g)	(g)	(g)	(g)	(mg)	(mg)
Breakfast							
Snack							
Lunch							
Snack							
Dinner							
Total Calories Consumed							

Daily Physical Activity_____

Daily Calories burned_____

Formula: (Calories consumed — Calories burned) =
Total calories intake per day

_____ = _____

Day #

Date:
Weight:
Time:
Water (oz):

Food description	Cals	F a t	C a r b s	F i b	P r o t	S o d	Ch o l
		(g)	(g)	(g)	(g)	(mg)	(mg)
Breakfast							
Snack							
Lunch							
Snack							
Dinner							
Total Calories Consumed							

Daily Physical Activity_____

Daily Calories burned_____

Formula: (Calories consumed — Calories burned) =
Total calories intake per day

_____ = _____

Day #   Date:
Weight:
Time:
Water (oz):

Food description	Cals	Fat	Carbs	Fib	Prot	Sod	Chol
		(g)	(g)	(g)	(g)	(mg)	(mg)
Breakfast							
Snack							
Lunch							
Snack							
Dinner							
Total Calories Consumed							

Daily Physical Activity_____

Daily Calories burned_____

**Formula: (Calories consumed — Calories burned) =
Total calories intake per day**

_____ = _____

Day # | Date:
Weight:
Time:
Water (oz):

Food description	Cals	F a t	C a r b s	F i b	P r o t	S o d	Ch o l
		(g)	(g)	(g)	(g)	(mg)	(mg)
Breakfast							
Snack							
Lunch							
Snack							
Dinner							
Total Calories Consumed							

Daily Physical Activity_____

Daily Calories burned_____

Formula: (Calories consumed — Calories burned) =
Total calories intake per day

_____ = _____

Day # | Date:
Weight:
Time:
Water (oz):

Food description	Cals	Fat (g)	Carbs (g)	Fib (g)	Prot (g)	Sod (mg)	Chol (mg)
Breakfast							
Snack							
Lunch							
Snack							
Dinner							
Total Calories Consumed							

Daily Physical Activity_____

Daily Calories burned_____
Formula: (Calories consumed — Calories burned) =
Total calories intake per day

_____ = _____

Day #	Date: Weight: Time: Water (oz):

Food description	Cals	F a t	C a r b s	F i b	P r o t	S o d	Ch o l
		(g)	(g)	(g)	(g)	(mg)	(mg)
Breakfast							
Snack							
Lunch							
Snack							
Dinner							
Total Calories Consumed							

Daily Physical Activity_____

Daily Calories burned_____

Formula: (Calories consumed — Calories burned) =
Total calories intake per day

_____ = _____

Day #   Date:
  Weight:
  Time:
  Water (oz):

Food description	Cals	Fat	Carbs	Fib	Prot	Sod	Chol
		(g)	(g)	(g)	(g)	(mg)	(mg)
Breakfast							
Snack							
Lunch							
Snack							
Dinner							
Total Calories Consumed							

Daily Physical Activity_____

Daily Calories burned_____

Formula: (Calories consumed — Calories burned) =
Total calories intake per day

_____ = _____

| Day # | Date:
Weight:
Time:
Water (oz): |

Food description	Cals	Fat	Carbs	Fib	Prot	Sod	Chol
		(g)	(g)	(g)	(g)	(mg)	(mg)
Breakfast							
Snack							
Lunch							
Snack							
Dinner							
Total Calories Consumed							

Daily Physical Activity_____

Daily Calories burned_____

Formula: (Calories consumed − Calories burned) =
Total calories intake per day

_____ = _____

Day #

Date:
Weight:
Time:
Water (oz):

Food description	Cals	Fat (g)	Carbs (g)	Fib (g)	Prot (g)	Sod (mg)	Chol (mg)
Breakfast							
Snack							
Lunch							
Snack							
Dinner							
Total Calories Consumed							

Daily Physical Activity_____

Daily Calories burned_____

Formula: (Calories consumed − Calories burned) =
Total calories intake per day

_____ = _____

Day # Date:
       Weight:
       Time:
       Water (oz):

Food description	Cals	Fat	Carbs	Fib	Prot	Sod	Chol
		(g)	(g)	(g)	(g)	(mg)	(mg)
Breakfast							
Snack							
Lunch							
Snack							
Dinner							
Total Calories Consumed							

Daily Physical Activity_____

Daily Calories burned_____

Formula: (Calories consumed — Calories burned) =
Total calories intake per day

_____ = _____

Day # | Date:
Weight:
Time:
Water (oz):

Food description	Cals	Fat	Carbs	Fib	Prot	Sod	Chol
		(g)	(g)	(g)	(g)	(mg)	(mg)
Breakfast							
Snack							
Lunch							
Snack							
Dinner							
Total Calories Consumed							

Daily Physical Activity_____

Daily Calories burned_____

Formula: (Calories consumed — Calories burned) =
Total calories intake per day

_____ = _____

Day #	Date: Weight: Time: Water (oz):

Food description	Cals	F a t	C a r b s	F i b	P r o t	S o d	Ch o l
		(g)	(g)	(g)	(g)	(mg)	(mg)
Breakfast							
Snack							
Lunch							
Snack							
Dinner							
Total Calories Consumed							

Daily Physical Activity_____

Daily Calories burned_____

**Formula: (Calories consumed — Calories burned) =
Total calories intake per day**

_____ = _____

Day #	Date:
	Weight:
	Time:
	Water (oz):

Food description	Cals	Fat	Carbs	Fib	Prot	Sod	Chol
		(g)	(g)	(g)	(g)	(mg)	(mg)
Breakfast							
Snack							
Lunch							
Snack							
Dinner							
Total Calories Consumed							

Daily Physical Activity_____

Daily Calories burned_____

Formula: (Calories consumed — Calories burned) =
Total calories intake per day

_____ = _____

Day # | Date:
Weight:
Time:
Water (oz):

Food description	Cals	F a t	C a r b s	F i b	P r o t	S o d	Ch o l
		(g)	(g)	(g)	(g)	(mg)	(mg)
Breakfast							
Snack							
Lunch							
Snack							
Dinner							
Total Calories Consumed							

Daily Physical Activity_____

Daily Calories burned_____

Formula: (Calories consumed — Calories burned) =
Total calories intake per day

_____ = _____

Day #

Date:
Weight:
Time:
Water (oz):

Food description	Cals	F a t (g)	C a r b s (g)	F i b (g)	P r o t (g)	S o d (mg)	Ch o l (mg)
Breakfast							
Snack							
Lunch							
Snack							
Dinner							
Total Calories Consumed							

Daily Physical Activity_____

Daily Calories burned_____

Formula: (Calories consumed — Calories burned) =
Total calories intake per day

_____ = _____

Day #   Date:
Weight:
Time:
Water (oz):

Food description	Cals	Fat (g)	Carbs (g)	Fib (g)	Prot (g)	Sod (mg)	Chol (mg)
Breakfast							
Snack							
Lunch							
Snack							
Dinner							
Total Calories Consumed							

Daily Physical Activity_____

Daily Calories burned_____
**Formula: (Calories consumed — Calories burned) =
Total calories intake per day**

_____ = _____

Day #
Date:
Weight:
Time:
Water (oz):

Food description	Cals	Fat	Carbs	Fib	Prot	Sod	Chol
		(g)	(g)	(g)	(g)	(mg)	(mg)
Breakfast							
Snack							
Lunch							
Snack							
Dinner							
Total Calories Consumed							

Daily Physical Activity_____

Daily Calories burned_____

Formula: (Calories consumed — Calories burned) =
Total calories intake per day

_____ = _____

Day #	Date: Weight: Time: Water (oz):

Food description	Cals	Fat	Carbs	Fib	Prot	Sod	Chol
		(g)	(g)	(g)	(g)	(mg)	(mg)
Breakfast							
Snack							
Lunch							
Snack							
Dinner							
Total Calories Consumed							

Daily Physical Activity_____

Daily Calories burned_____

Formula: (Calories consumed — Calories burned) =
Total calories intake per day

_____ = _____

Day # | Date:
Weight:
Time:
Water (oz):

Food description	Cals	Fat	Carbs	Fib	Prot	Sod	Chol
		(g)	(g)	(g)	(g)	(mg)	(mg)
Breakfast							
Snack							
Lunch							
Snack							
Dinner							
Total Calories Consumed							

Daily Physical Activity_____

Daily Calories burned_____

Formula: (Calories consumed − Calories burned) =
Total calories intake per day

_____ = _____

Day #

Date:
Weight:
Time:
Water (oz):

Food description	Cals	F a t	C a r b s	F i b	P r o t	S o d	Ch o l
		(g)	(g)	(g)	(g)	(mg)	(mg)
Breakfast							
Snack							
Lunch							
Snack							
Dinner							
Total Calories Consumed							

Daily Physical Activity_____

Daily Calories burned_____

Formula: (Calories consumed — Calories burned) =
Total calories intake per day

_____ = _____

Day #   Date:
Weight:
Time:
Water (oz):

Food description	Cals	Fat	Carbs	Fib	Prot	Sod	Chol
		(g)	(g)	(g)	(g)	(mg)	(mg)
Breakfast							
Snack							
Lunch							
Snack							
Dinner							
Total Calories Consumed							

Daily Physical Activity_____

Daily Calories burned_____

Formula: (Calories consumed — Calories burned) =
Total calories intake per day

_____ = _____

Day #   Date:
Weight:
Time:
Water (oz):

Food description	Cals	F a t (g)	C a r b s (g)	F i b (g)	P r o t (g)	S o d (mg)	Ch o l (mg)
Breakfast							
Snack							
Lunch							
Snack							
Dinner							
Total Calories Consumed							

Daily Physical Activity_____

Daily Calories burned_____

Formula: (Calories consumed — Calories burned) =
Total calories intake per day

_____ = _____

Day #   **Date:**
Weight:
Time:
Water (oz):

Food description	Cals	Fat	Carbs	Fib	Prot	Sod	Chol
		(g)	(g)	(g)	(g)	(mg)	(mg)
Breakfast							
Snack							
Lunch							
Snack							
Dinner							
Total Calories Consumed							

Daily Physical Activity_____

Daily Calories burned_____

Formula: (Calories consumed — Calories burned) =
Total calories intake per day

_____ = _____

Day # | Date:
Weight:
Time:
Water (oz):

Food description	Cals	F a t	C a r b s	F i b	P r o t	S o d	Ch o l
		(g)	(g)	(g)	(g)	(mg)	(mg)
Breakfast							
Snack							
Lunch							
Snack							
Dinner							
Total Calories Consumed							

Daily Physical Activity_____

Daily Calories burned_____

**Formula: (Calories consumed — Calories burned) =
Total calories intake per day**

_____ = _____

Day # | Date:
Weight:
Time:
Water (oz):

Food description	Cals	F a t	C a r b s	F i b	P r o t	S o d	Ch o l
		(g)	(g)	(g)	(g)	(mg)	(mg)
Breakfast							
Snack							
Lunch							
Snack							
Dinner							
Total Calories Consumed							

Daily Physical Activity_____

Daily Calories burned_____

Formula: (Calories consumed − Calories burned) =
Total calories intake per day

_____ = _____

Day #   Date:
Weight:
Time:
Water (oz):

Food description	Cals	F a t (g)	C a r b s (g)	F i b (g)	P r o t (g)	S o d (mg)	Ch o l (mg)
Breakfast							
Snack							
Lunch							
Snack							
Dinner							
Total Calories Consumed							

Daily Physical Activity_____

Daily Calories burned_____

Formula: (Calories consumed — Calories burned) =
Total calories intake per day

_____ = _____

Day #   Date:
         Weight:
         Time:
         Water (oz):

Food description	Cals	Fat	Carbs	Fib	Prot	Sod	Chol
		(g)	(g)	(g)	(g)	(mg)	(mg)
Breakfast							
Snack							
Lunch							
Snack							
Dinner							
Total Calories Consumed							

Daily Physical Activity_____

Daily Calories burned_____

Formula: (Calories consumed — Calories burned) =
Total calories intake per day

_____ = _____

Day #	Date: Weight: Time: Water (oz):

Food description	Cals	Fat	Carbs	Fib	Prot	Sod	Chol
		(g)	(g)	(g)	(g)	(mg)	(mg)
Breakfast							
Snack							
Lunch							
Snack							
Dinner							
Total Calories Consumed							

Daily Physical Activity_____

Daily Calories burned_____

Formula: (Calories consumed — Calories burned) =
Total calories intake per day

_____ = _____

Day #
Date:
Weight:
Time:
Water (oz):

Food description	Cals	Fat	Carbs	Fib	Prot	Sod	Chol
		(g)	(g)	(g)	(g)	(mg)	(mg)
Breakfast							
Snack							
Lunch							
Snack							
Dinner							
Total Calories Consumed							

Daily Physical Activity_____

Daily Calories burned_____

Formula: (Calories consumed — Calories burned) =
Total calories intake per day

_____ = _____

| Day # | Date:
Weight:
Time:
Water (oz): |

Food description	Cals	F a t	C a r b s	F i b	P r o t	S o d	Ch o l
		(g)	(g)	(g)	(g)	(mg)	(mg)
Breakfast							
Snack							
Lunch							
Snack							
Dinner							
Total Calories Consumed							

Daily Physical Activity_____

Daily Calories burned_____

**Formula: (Calories consumed — Calories burned) =
Total calories intake per day**

_____ = _____

Day #	Date: Weight: Time: Water (oz):

Food description	Cals	F a t	C a r b s	F i b	P r o t	S o d	Ch o l
		(g)	(g)	(g)	(g)	(mg)	(mg)
Breakfast							
Snack							
Lunch							
Snack							
Dinner							
Total Calories Consumed							

Daily Physical Activity_____

Daily Calories burned_____

Formula: (Calories consumed − Calories burned) =
Total calories intake per day

_____ = _____

Day #	Date: Weight: Time: Water (oz):

Food description	Cals	F a t	C a r b s	F i b	P r o t	S o d	Ch o l
		(g)	(g)	(g)	(g)	(mg)	(mg)
Breakfast							
Snack							
Lunch							
Snack							
Dinner							
Total Calories Consumed							

Daily Physical Activity_____

Daily Calories burned_____

Formula: (Calories consumed − Calories burned) =
Total calories intake per day

_____ = _____

Day #

Date:
Weight:
Time:
Water (oz):

Food description	Cals	F a t	C a r b s	F i b	P r o t	S o d	Ch o l
		(g)	(g)	(g)	(g)	(mg)	(mg)
Breakfast							
Snack							
Lunch							
Snack							
Dinner							
Total Calories Consumed							

Daily Physical Activity_____

Daily Calories burned_____

Formula: (Calories consumed — Calories burned) =
Total calories intake per day

_____ = _____

Day #   Date:
        Weight:
        Time:
        Water (oz):

Food description	Cals	Fat	Carbs	Fib	Prot	Sod	Chol
		(g)	(g)	(g)	(g)	(mg)	(mg)
Breakfast							
Snack							
Lunch							
Snack							
Dinner							
Total Calories Consumed							

Daily Physical Activity_____

Daily Calories burned_____

Formula: (Calories consumed — Calories burned) =
Total calories intake per day

_____ = _____

Day #

Date:
Weight:
Time:
Water (oz):

Food description	Cals	Fat	Carbs	Fib	Prot	Sod	Chol
		(g)	(g)	(g)	(g)	(mg)	(mg)
Breakfast							
Snack							
Lunch							
Snack							
Dinner							
Total Calories Consumed							

Daily Physical Activity_____

Daily Calories burned_____

Formula: (Calories consumed — Calories burned) =
Total calories intake per day

_____ = _____

Day #	Date: Weight: Time: Water (oz):

Food description	Cals	Fat	Carbs	Fib	Prot	Sod	Chol
		(g)	(g)	(g)	(g)	(mg)	(mg)
Breakfast							
Snack							
Lunch							
Snack							
Dinner							
Total Calories Consumed							

Daily Physical Activity_____

Daily Calories burned_____

Formula: (Calories consumed — Calories burned) =
Total calories intake per day

_____ = _____

Day #

Date:
Weight:
Time:
Water (oz):

Food description	Cals	Fat	Carbs	Fib	Prot	Sod	Chol
		(g)	(g)	(g)	(g)	(mg)	(mg)
Breakfast							
Snack							
Lunch							
Snack							
Dinner							
Total Calories Consumed							

Daily Physical Activity_____

Daily Calories burned_____

Formula: (Calories consumed — Calories burned) =
Total calories intake per day

_____ = _____

Day #   Date:
      Weight:
      Time:
      Water (oz):

Food description	Cals	Fat	Carbs	Fib	Prot	Sod	Chol
		(g)	(g)	(g)	(g)	(mg)	(mg)
Breakfast							
Snack							
Lunch							
Snack							
Dinner							
Total Calories Consumed							

Daily Physical Activity_____

Daily Calories burned_____

Formula: (Calories consumed — Calories burned) =
Total calories intake per day

_____ = _____

Day #
Date:
Weight:
Time:
Water (oz):

Food description	Cals	Fat	Carbs	Fib	Prot	Sod	Chol
		(g)	(g)	(g)	(g)	(mg)	(mg)
Breakfast							
Snack							
Lunch							
Snack							
Dinner							
Total Calories Consumed							

Daily Physical Activity_____

Daily Calories burned_____

Formula: (Calories consumed — Calories burned) =
Total calories intake per day

_____ = _____

Day # | Date:
Weight:
Time:
Water (oz):

Food description	Cals	F a t	C a r b s	F i b	P r o t	S o d	Ch o l
		(g)	(g)	(g)	(g)	(mg)	(mg)
Breakfast							
Snack							
Lunch							
Snack							
Dinner							
Total Calories Consumed							

Daily Physical Activity_____

Daily Calories burned_____

Formula: (Calories consumed — Calories burned) =
Total calories intake per day

_____ = _____

Day # Date:
Weight:
Time:
Water (oz):

Food description	Cals	Fat (g)	Carbs (g)	Fib (g)	Prot (g)	Sod (mg)	Chol (mg)
Breakfast							
Snack							
Lunch							
Snack							
Dinner							
Total Calories Consumed							

Daily Physical Activity_____

Daily Calories burned_____

Formula: (Calories consumed — Calories burned) =
Total calories intake per day

_____ = _____

| Day # | Date:
Weight:
Time:
Water (oz): |

Food description	Cals	Fat (g)	Carbs (g)	Fib (g)	Prot (g)	Sod (mg)	Chol (mg)
Breakfast							
Snack							
Lunch							
Snack							
Dinner							
Total Calories Consumed							

Daily Physical Activity_____

Daily Calories burned_____

Formula: (Calories consumed — Calories burned) =
Total calories intake per day

_____ = _____

Day # | Date:
Weight:
Time:
Water (oz):

Food description	Cals	F a t	C a r b s	F i b	P r o t	S o d	Ch o l
		(g)	(g)	(g)	(g)	(mg)	(mg)
Breakfast							
Snack							
Lunch							
Snack							
Dinner							
Total Calories Consumed							

Daily Physical Activity_____

Daily Calories burned_____

Formula: (Calories consumed − Calories burned) =
Total calories intake per day

_____ = _____

Day #	Date: Weight: Time: Water (oz):

Food description	Cals	Fat	Carbs	Fib	Prot	Sod	Chol
		(g)	(g)	(g)	(g)	(mg)	(mg)
Breakfast							
Snack							
Lunch							
Snack							
Dinner							
Total Calories Consumed							

Daily Physical Activity_____

Daily Calories burned_____

Formula: (Calories consumed — Calories burned) =
Total calories intake per day

_____ = _____

Day #

Date:
Weight:
Time:
Water (oz):

Food description	Cals	F a t	C a r b s	F i b	P r o t	S o d	Ch o l
		(g)	(g)	(g)	(g)	(mg)	(mg)
Breakfast							
Snack							
Lunch							
Snack							
Dinner							
Total Calories Consumed							

Daily Physical Activity_____

Daily Calories burned_____

Formula: (Calories consumed — Calories burned) =
Total calories intake per day

_____ = _____

Day #   Date:
Weight:
Time:
Water (oz):

Food description	Cals	F a t (g)	C a r b s (g)	F i b (g)	P r o t (g)	S o d (mg)	Ch o l (mg)
Breakfast							
Snack							
Lunch							
Snack							
Dinner							
Total Calories Consumed							

Daily Physical Activity_____

Daily Calories burned_____

Formula: (Calories consumed — Calories burned) =
Total calories intake per day

_____ = _____

Day #	Date: Weight: Time: Water (oz):

Food description	Cals	Fat	Carbs	Fib	Prot	Sod	Chol
		(g)	(g)	(g)	(g)	(mg)	(mg)
Breakfast							
Snack							
Lunch							
Snack							
Dinner							
Total Calories Consumed							

Daily Physical Activity_____

Daily Calories burned_____

Formula: (Calories consumed — Calories burned) =
Total calories intake per day

_____ = _____

Day #	Date: Weight: Time: Water (oz):

Food description	Cals	F a t	C a r b s	F i b	P r o t	S o d	Ch o l
		(g)	(g)	(g)	(g)	(mg)	(mg)
Breakfast							
Snack							
Lunch							
Snack							
Dinner							
Total Calories Consumed							

Daily Physical Activity_____

Daily Calories burned_____

Formula: (Calories consumed — Calories burned) =
Total calories intake per day

_____ = _____

Day #

Date:
Weight:
Time:
Water (oz):

Food description	Cals	F a t	C a r b s	F i b	P r o t	S o d	Ch o l
		(g)	(g)	(g)	(g)	(mg)	(mg)
Breakfast							
Snack							
Lunch							
Snack							
Dinner							
Total Calories Consumed							

Daily Physical Activity_____

Daily Calories burned_____

Formula: (Calories consumed − Calories burned) =
Total calories intake per day

_____ = _____

Day # | Date:
Weight:
Time:
Water (oz):

Food description	Cals	F a t (g)	C a r b s (g)	F i b (g)	P r o t (g)	S o d (mg)	Ch o l (mg)
Breakfast							
Snack							
Lunch							
Snack							
Dinner							
Total Calories Consumed							

Daily Physical Activity_____

Daily Calories burned_____

Formula: (Calories consumed — Calories burned) =
Total calories intake per day

_____ = _____

Day #

Date:
Weight:
Time:
Water (oz):

Food description	Cals	F a t	C a r b s	F i b	P r o t	S o d	Ch o l
		(g)	(g)	(g)	(g)	(mg)	(mg)
Breakfast							
Snack							
Lunch							
Snack							
Dinner							
Total Calories Consumed							

Daily Physical Activity_____

Daily Calories burned_____

Formula: (Calories consumed — Calories burned) =
Total calories intake per day

_____ = _____

Day # | Date:
Weight:
Time:
Water (oz):

Food description	Cals	F a t	C a r b s	F i b	P r o t	S o d	Ch o l
		(g)	(g)	(g)	(g)	(mg)	(mg)
Breakfast							
Snack							
Lunch							
Snack							
Dinner							
Total Calories Consumed							

Daily Physical Activity_____

Daily Calories burned_____
Formula: (Calories consumed — Calories burned) =
Total calories intake per day

_____ = _____

Day # | Date:
Weight:
Time:
Water (oz):

Food description	Cals	Fat	Carbs	Fib	Prot	Sod	Chol
		(g)	(g)	(g)	(g)	(mg)	(mg)
Breakfast							
Snack							
Lunch							
Snack							
Dinner							
Total Calories Consumed							

Daily Physical Activity_____

Daily Calories burned_____

Formula: (Calories consumed — Calories burned) =
Total calories intake per day

_____ = _____

Day #	Date:
	Weight:
	Time:
	Water (oz):

Food description	Cals	F a t	C a r b s	F i b	P r o t	S o d	Ch o l
		(g)	(g)	(g)	(g)	(mg)	(mg)
Breakfast							
Snack							
Lunch							
Snack							
Dinner							
Total Calories Consumed							

Daily Physical Activity_____

Daily Calories burned_____

Formula: (Calories consumed — Calories burned) =
Total calories intake per day

_____ = _____

Day
#

Date:
Weight:
Time:
Water (oz):

Food description	Cals	F a t	C a r b s	F i b	P r o t	S o d	Ch o l
		(g)	(g)	(g)	(g)	(mg)	(mg)
Breakfast							
Snack							
Lunch							
Snack							
Dinner							
Total Calories Consumed							

Daily Physical Activity_____

Daily Calories burned_____

Formula: (Calories consumed — Calories burned) =
Total calories intake per day

_____ = _____

Day # — Date:
Weight:
Time:
Water (oz):

Food description	Cals	F a t	C a r b s	F i b	P r o t	S o d	Ch o l
		(g)	(g)	(g)	(g)	(mg)	(mg)
Breakfast							
Snack							
Lunch							
Snack							
Dinner							
Total Calories Consumed							

Daily Physical Activity_____

Daily Calories burned_____

Formula: (Calories consumed — Calories burned) =
Total calories intake per day

_____ = _____

Day #   Date:
Weight:
Time:
Water (oz):

Food description	Cals	Fat (g)	Carbs (g)	Fib (g)	Prot (g)	Sod (mg)	Chol (mg)
Breakfast							
Snack							
Lunch							
Snack							
Dinner							
Total Calories Consumed							

Daily Physical Activity_____

Daily Calories burned_____

Formula: (Calories consumed — Calories burned) =
Total calories intake per day

_____ = _____

Day #   Date:
Weight:
Time:
Water (oz):

Food description	Cals	F a t	C a r b s	F i b	P r o t	S o d	Ch o l
		(g)	(g)	(g)	(g)	(mg)	(mg)
Breakfast							
Snack							
Lunch							
Snack							
Dinner							
Total Calories Consumed							

Daily Physical Activity_____

Daily Calories burned_____

Formula: (Calories consumed — Calories burned) =
Total calories intake per day

_____ = _____

Day #
Date:
Weight:
Time:
Water (oz):

Food description	Cals	Fat	Carbs	Fib	Prot	Sod	Chol
		(g)	(g)	(g)	(g)	(mg)	(mg)
Breakfast							
Snack							
Lunch							
Snack							
Dinner							
Total Calories Consumed							

Daily Physical Activity_____

Daily Calories burned_____

Formula: (Calories consumed — Calories burned) =
Total calories intake per day

_____ = _____

Day # | Date:
Weight:
Time:
Water (oz):

Food description	Cals	F a t	C a r b s	F i b	P r o t	S o d	Ch o l
		(g)	(g)	(g)	(g)	(mg)	(mg)
Breakfast							
Snack							
Lunch							
Snack							
Dinner							
Total Calories Consumed							

Daily Physical Activity_____

Daily Calories burned_____

Formula: (Calories consumed — Calories burned) =
Total calories intake per day

_____ = _____

Day # | Date:
Weight:
Time:
Water (oz):

Food description	Cals	F a t	C a r b s	F i b	P r o t	S o d	Ch o l
		(g)	(g)	(g)	(g)	(mg)	(mg)
Breakfast							
Snack							
Lunch							
Snack							
Dinner							
Total Calories Consumed							

Daily Physical Activity_____

Daily Calories burned_____

**Formula: (Calories consumed − Calories burned) =
Total calories intake per day**

_____ = _____

Day #	Date: Weight: Time: Water (oz):

Food description	Cals	F a t	C a r b s	F i b	P r o t	S o d	Ch o l
		(g)	(g)	(g)	(g)	(mg)	(mg)
Breakfast							
Snack							
Lunch							
Snack							
Dinner							
Total Calories Consumed							

Daily Physical Activity_____

Daily Calories burned_____

Formula: (Calories consumed — Calories burned) =
Total calories intake per day

_____ = _____

Day #   Date:
         Weight:
         Time:
         Water (oz):

Food description	Cals	F a t	C a r b s	F i b	P r o t	S o d	Ch o l
		(g)	(g)	(g)	(g)	(mg)	(mg)
Breakfast							
Snack							
Lunch							
Snack							
Dinner							
Total Calories Consumed							

Daily Physical Activity_____

Daily Calories burned_____

Formula: (Calories consumed — Calories burned) =
Total calories intake per day

_____ = _____

Day #	Date: Weight: Time: Water (oz):

Food description	Cals	F a t	C a r b s	F i b	P r o t	S o d	Ch o l
		(g)	(g)	(g)	(g)	(mg)	(mg)
Breakfast							
Snack							
Lunch							
Snack							
Dinner							
Total Calories Consumed							

Daily Physical Activity_____

Daily Calories burned_____

Formula: (Calories consumed — Calories burned) =
Total calories intake per day

_____ = _____

Day # Date:
Weight:
Time:
Water (oz):

Food description	Cals	Fat	Carbs	Fib	Prot	Sod	Chol
		(g)	(g)	(g)	(g)	(mg)	(mg)
Breakfast							
Snack							
Lunch							
Snack							
Dinner							
Total Calories Consumed							

Daily Physical Activity_____

Daily Calories burned_____

**Formula: (Calories consumed — Calories burned) =
Total calories intake per day**

_____ = _____

Day #	Date: Weight: Time: Water (oz):

Food description	Cals	F a t (g)	C a r b s (g)	F i b (g)	P r o t (g)	S o d (mg)	Ch o l (mg)
Breakfast							
Snack							
Lunch							
Snack							
Dinner							
Total Calories Consumed							

Daily Physical Activity_____

Daily Calories burned_____

Formula: (Calories consumed — Calories burned) =
Total calories intake per day

_____ = _____

Day #   Date:
  Weight:
  Time:
  Water (oz):

Food description	Cals	Fat (g)	Carbs (g)	Fib (g)	Prot (g)	Sod (mg)	Chol (mg)
Breakfast							
Snack							
Lunch							
Snack							
Dinner							
Total Calories Consumed							

Daily Physical Activity_____

Daily Calories burned_____
Formula: (Calories consumed — Calories burned) =
Total calories intake per day

_____ = _____

Day #	Date:
	Weight:
	Time:
	Water (oz):

Food description	Cals	F a t (g)	C a r b s (g)	F i b (g)	P r o t (g)	S o d (mg)	Ch o l (mg)
Breakfast							
Snack							
Lunch							
Snack							
Dinner							
Total Calories Consumed							

Daily Physical Activity_____

Daily Calories burned_____

Formula: (Calories consumed — Calories burned) =
Total calories intake per day

_____ = _____

Day # Date:
Weight:
Time:
Water (oz):

Food description	Cals	Fat	Carbs	Fib	Prot	Sod	Chol
		(g)	(g)	(g)	(g)	(mg)	(mg)
Breakfast							
Snack							
Lunch							
Snack							
Dinner							
Total Calories Consumed							

Daily Physical Activity_____

Daily Calories burned_____

Formula: (Calories consumed − Calories burned) =
Total calories intake per day

_____ = _____

Day
#

Date:
Weight:
Time:
Water (oz):

Food description	Cals	Fat	Carbs	Fib	Prot	Sod	Chol
		(g)	(g)	(g)	(g)	(mg)	(mg)
Breakfast							
Snack							
Lunch							
Snack							
Dinner							
Total Calories Consumed							

Daily Physical Activity_____

Daily Calories burned_____

Formula: (Calories consumed — Calories burned) =
Total calories intake per day

_____ = _____

Day # Date:
Weight:
Time:
Water (oz):

Food description	Cals	Fat	Carbs	Fib	Prot	Sod	Chol
		(g)	(g)	(g)	(g)	(mg)	(mg)
Breakfast							
Snack							
Lunch							
Snack							
Dinner							
Total Calories Consumed							

Daily Physical Activity_____

Daily Calories burned_____

Formula: (Calories consumed — Calories burned) =
Total calories intake per day

_____ = _____

Day #	Date: Weight: Time: Water (oz):

Food description	Cals	F a t	C a r b s	F i b	P r o t	S o d	Ch o l
		(g)	(g)	(g)	(g)	(mg)	(mg)
Breakfast							
Snack							
Lunch							
Snack							
Dinner							
Total Calories Consumed							

Daily Physical Activity_____

Daily Calories burned_____

Formula: (Calories consumed — Calories burned) =
Total calories intake per day

_____ = _____

Day # | Date:
Weight:
Time:
Water (oz):

Food description	Cals	F a t	C a r b s	F i b	P r o t	S o d	Ch o l
		(g)	(g)	(g)	(g)	(mg)	(mg)
Breakfast							
Snack							
Lunch							
Snack							
Dinner							
Total Calories Consumed							

Daily Physical Activity_____

Daily Calories burned_____

Formula: (Calories consumed − Calories burned) =
Total calories intake per day

_____ = _____

Day # Date: Weight: Time: Water (oz):

Food description	Cals	Fat (g)	Carbs (g)	Fib (g)	Prot (g)	Sod (mg)	Chol (mg)
Breakfast							
Snack							
Lunch							
Snack							
Dinner							
Total Calories Consumed							

Daily Physical Activity_____

Daily Calories burned_____

Formula: (Calories consumed — Calories burned) =
Total calories intake per day

_____ = _____

Day #   Date:
Weight:
Time:
Water (oz):

Food description	Cals	Fat (g)	Carbs (g)	Fib (g)	Prot (g)	Sod (mg)	Chol (mg)
Breakfast							
Snack							
Lunch							
Snack							
Dinner							
Total Calories Consumed							

Daily Physical Activity_____

Daily Calories burned_____

Formula: (Calories consumed − Calories burned) =
Total calories intake per day

_____ = _____

Day #   Date:
Weight:
Time:
Water (oz):

Food description	Cals	Fat (g)	Carbs (g)	Fib (g)	Prot (g)	Sod (mg)	Chol (mg)
Breakfast							
Snack							
Lunch							
Snack							
Dinner							
Total Calories Consumed							

Daily Physical Activity_____

Daily Calories burned_____

Formula: (Calories consumed — Calories burned) =
Total calories intake per day

_____ = _____

Day #	Date: Weight: Time: Water (oz):

Food description	Cals	Fat	Carbs	Fib	Prot	Sod	Chol
		(g)	(g)	(g)	(g)	(mg)	(mg)
Breakfast							
Snack							
Lunch							
Snack							
Dinner							
Total Calories Consumed							

Daily Physical Activity_____

Daily Calories burned_____

Formula: (Calories consumed — Calories burned) =
Total calories intake per day

_____ = _____

Day #

Date:
Weight:
Time:
Water (oz):

Food description	Cals	Fat	Carbs	Fib	Prot	Sod	Chol
		(g)	(g)	(g)	(g)	(mg)	(mg)
Breakfast							
Snack							
Lunch							
Snack							
Dinner							
Total Calories Consumed							

Daily Physical Activity_____

Daily Calories burned_____

Formula: (Calories consumed — Calories burned) =
Total calories intake per day

_____ = _____

Day # **Date:**
Weight:
Time:
Water (oz):

Food description	Cals	Fat	Carbs	Fib	Prot	Sod	Chol
		(g)	(g)	(g)	(g)	(mg)	(mg)
Breakfast							
Snack							
Lunch							
Snack							
Dinner							
Total Calories Consumed							

Daily Physical Activity_____

Daily Calories burned_____

Formula: (Calories consumed — Calories burned) =
Total calories intake per day

_____ = _____

Day #   Date:
         Weight:
         Time:
         Water (oz):

Food description	Cals	F a t (g)	C a r b s (g)	F i b (g)	P r o t (g)	S o d (mg)	Ch o l (mg)
Breakfast							
Snack							
Lunch							
Snack							
Dinner							
Total Calories Consumed							

Daily Physical Activity_____

Daily Calories burned_____

Formula: (Calories consumed — Calories burned) =
Total calories intake per day

_____ = _____

APPENDIX A

TABLE OF PERCENTAGES ACCORDING TO THE USDA

	% Carbs	% Prot	% Fat
SAFE RATIOS	45% TO 65%	10% TO 35%	20% TO 35%

APPENDIX B

BODY FAT %

	WOMEN	MAN
ESSENTIAL FAT	10 – 13%	2 – 5%
ATHLETES	14 – 20%	6 – 13 %
FITNESS	21 – 24%	14 – 17%
AVERAGE	25 – 31 %	18 – 24%
OBESE	32% +	25% +

APPENDIX C

TYPES OF NUTRIENTS (MACROMOLECULES) IN FOOD

MACROMOLECULE	STRUCTURE	FUNCTIONS IN BODY
Carbohydrates	Polymer made from units of mono-saccharides	-Source of carbon for building other organic compounds -Immediate fuel source
Fats/Lipids	Made of fatty acids and glycerol units (monomers)	-Major important role in cellular membranes -Fuel source
Proteins	Chains of amino acids.	Source of raw material for the production enzymes and proteins.
Vitamins	Small organic molecules.	-Variety of functions. -Helps enzymes.
Minerals	Ionic and inorganic.	Some minerals have a diverse function when they bond with organic molecules
Water	Inorganic molecule.	Major component of cells and body fluids

APPENDIX D

LIST OF SOME VITAMINS AND THEIR ROLE IN OUR HEALTH

SOME VITAMINS	MAJOR FOOD SOURCES	FUNCTIONS IN BODY
Vitamin B1	In pork, legumes, peanuts, whole grains	In carbohydrate use Nervous system function
Vitamin B2	In dairy, meats, whole grains, vegetables	Use in carbohydrates, proteins and for the metabolism of fat.
Niacin	In nuts, meats, grains, legumes	In energy metabolism
Vitamin B6	In meats, vegetables, whole grains	In protein, fat and carbohydrate metabolism
Pantothenic acid	In meats, dairy, whole grains	In energy metabolism and steroid production
Folic acid	In green vegetables, oranges, nuts, legumes	In energy metabolism and steroid production
Vitamin B12	In meats, eggs, dairy products	In the function of the nervous system and red blood cell production
Biotin	In legumes, other vegetables, meats	In energy metabolism
Vitamin C	In citrus, broccoli, green peppers	In bones, teeth, and skin growth and maintenance
Vitamin A	In green and orange	In skin, bones, teeth and hair, vision
Vitamin D	In fortified milk, egg yolks	In bones and teeth, calcium, phosphorous use.
Vitamin E	Seeds	certain toxins
Vitamin K	In green vegetables	In blood clotting

APPENDIX E

LIST OF SOME MINERALS AND THEIR ROLE IN OUR HEALTH

MINERAL	FOOD SOURCES	BODILY FUNCTIONS(SOME)
Calcium	In dairy, dark green vegetables, legumes	In bones and teeth, blood clotting, nerve and muscle function
Phosphorous	In dairy, meats, and grains	In bones and teeth. Also, in ATP production
Potassium	In meats, dairy, fruits, vegetables, and grains	In water balance, nerve and muscle function
Iodine	In Seafood, dairy, and iodized salt	In certain hormonal function
Zinc	In meats, seafood and grains	Helps digestive enzymes
Sulfur	In proteins from different foods	In the production of protein and cartilage
Iron	In meats, leafy vegetables, eggs, legumes and grains	Major role in hemoglobin

APPENDIX F

"Food+pyramid - Google Search." Food+pyramid - Google Search. N.p., n.d. Web. 13 Apr. 2016.

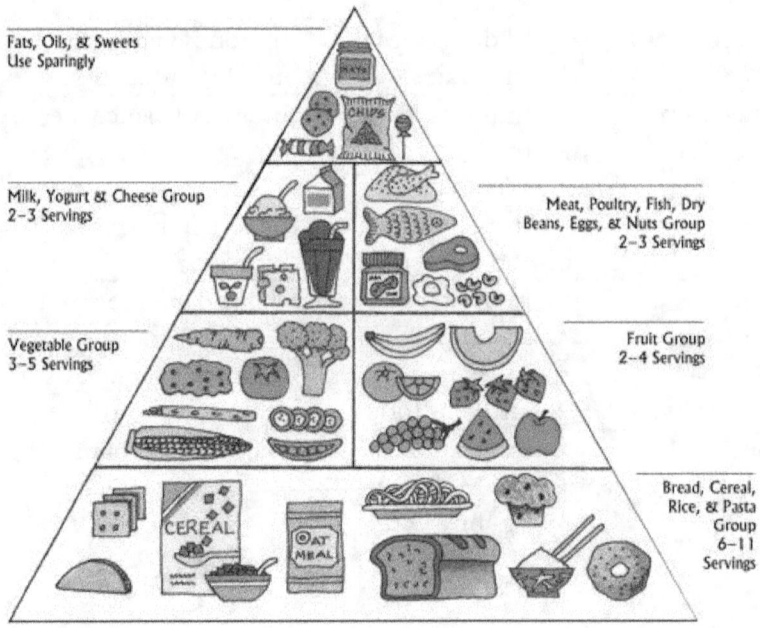

APPENDIX G

SAMPLE LOG BASED ON 130lbs, 1,690 Cal., 208 g Carbs, 130 grams of protein and 38 grams of fat. (sodium and cholesterol must be added)

Food Description	Cals	Carbs (g)	Fib (g)	Prot (g)
2 Scoops of Protein shake	320	4.00	6.00	60
½ cup of strawberries	24.00	4.10	1.40	0.50
2 slice of bread with 4 egg whites	200	16.00	4.00	28.00
7 dried nectarines	100.00	22.00	2.00	0
2 cups of coffee	4.00	0.20	0	0.30
1 tbsp. of fat free coffee cream	25.00	5.00	0	0
1 cup of rice	160.00	34.00	2.00	3.00
TOTAL 1	833.00	85.30	15.40	91.80
2 oz. of chicken	80.00	0	0	15.00
7 multigrain crackers	65.00	9.00	1.50	1.50
1 tangerine	70.00	17.00	2.00	0.50
2 cups of coffee	4.00	0.20	0	0.30

1 tbsp. of cream	25.00	5.00	0	0
TOTAL 2	1,077.00	116.50	18.90	109.10
1 small cinnamon roll	108.00	16.00	1.00	2.00
1 cup of rice	160.00	34.00	2.00	3.00
2 oz. of chicken	80.00	0	0	15.00
2/3 cup green beans	30.00	6.00	3.00	1.00
¼ cup of lentils	90.00	9.00	3.00	1.00
6 prunes	120	23.00	3.00	0.12
TOTAL 3	1,665.00	204.50	30.90	131.22
NOTES	GOAL ACHIEVED			

APPENDIX H
NUTRITIONAL VALUES QUICK REFERENCE GUIDE
"Cross-Reference Chart". Evaluating Research Methods in Psychology(n.d.): 158-59. Web.

NUTRITIONAL VALUES QUICK REFERENCE CHART

LEAN PROTEINS

Food Item	Qty	Calories	Protein	Carbs	Fat
Chicken Breast, skinless	4 oz	196	35.1	0	5.1
Turkey Breast, skinless	4 oz	178	33.9	0	3.7
Beef, ground extra lean	4 oz	265	21.1	0	19.3
Beef, top sirloin	4 oz	229	34.4	0	9.1
Beef, top Round	4 oz	214	35.9	0	6.7
Tuna, water packed	4 oz	120	26	0	1.0
Salmon, Atlantic	4 oz	206	28.8	0	9.2
Swordfish	4 oz	176	28.8	0	5.8
Cod	4 oz	119	25.9	0	1.0
Lobster	4 oz	111	23.2	1.5	0.7
Shrimp	4 oz	120	23	1	2.0
Protein Powder, Whey	2 scoops	180	35	4	3.0
Egg whites	6	102	21	1.8	0.0
Egg, whole	1	75	6.3	0.6	5.0
Turkey, Grnd, extra lean	4 oz	120	28	0	1.0

FRUIT

Food Item	Qty	Cal	Protein	Carbs	Fat
Apples	1	81	0.3	21.1	0.5
Banana	1	105	1.2	26.7	0.6
Cantaloupe	1/2	94	2.3	22.3	0.7
Grapefruit	1/2	46	0.6	11.9	0.1
Grapes (seedless)	10	36	0.3	8.9	0.3
Jelly, all fruit (no sugar)	2 tbsp	80	0	20	0
Nectarine	1	67	1.3	16	0.6
Peach	1	37	0.6	9.7	0.1
Pear	1	98	0.7	25.1	0.7
Plum	1	36	0.5	8.6	0.4
Orange	1	65	1.4	16.3	0.1
Orange Juice	8 fl oz	110	0.5	27	0
Raisins	1/4 cup	130	1.0	31	0.5
Raspberries	1 cup	62	1.2	14.2	0.6
Strawberries	1 cup	46	1.0	10.4	0.6
Watermelon (diced)	1 cup	50	1.0	3.6	0.2

COMPLEX CARBS (STARCHY)

Food Item	Qty	Calories	Protein	Carbs	Fat
Bagel, plain, whole wheat	1	150	6	33	1
Bread, whole wheat	1 slice	80	2.5	14	1
Bread, rye	1 slice	80	3	16	1
Potato, white	1 lg (8oz)	210	4.4	49	0.2
Potato, sweet	4 oz	136	2.1	31.6	0.4
Oatmeal, old-fashioned	1/3 c unckd	100	5	16	2
Cream of Rice	1/4 c unckd	170	3	38	0
Cream of Wheat	1 oz/1 pckt	100	3	21	1
Lentils	1/2 c ckd	115	9	20	0
Black eye peas	1/2 c boild	99	6.6	17.7	0.4
Pita, Whole wheat	1	170	6	35	2
Beans, Kidney	1/3 c ckd	75	5.1	13.5	0.3
Pasta, whole grain spelt	1 oz (dry)	95	4	20	0.7
Pasta, whole wheat	1 oz (dry)	105	4.5	20	1
Rice, Brown, "success"	1 c cooked	150	4	40	0
Rice, Wild	1 c cooked	166	6.5	35	0.6
Shredded Wheat	1 cup	144	3.6	33.4	1.4
Kashi cereal	3/4 cup	120	8	26	1
Yam	6 oz	180	4	41	0.2

COMPLEX CARBS (FIBROUS)

Food Item	Qty	Calories	Protein	Carbs	Fat
Asparagus	10 spears	40	4	6	0
Broccoli	1 cup	46	4.6	8.6	0.4
Brussel sprouts, boiled	1 cup	60	4	11.0	0.1
Cauliflower	1 cup	60	4.8	13.8	0.8
Carrots	1	31	0.8	7.3	0.1
Collard Greens	2 cups	36	1.6	8	0.4
Corn	1/2 cup	89	2.7	20.6	1.1
Cucumber	1 cup	16	0.8	3	0.2
Green Pepper	1 cup	24	0	6	0
Green Beans	6 oz	50	2	12	0
Kale	2 cups	56	4	11.8	0.8
Lettuce	2 cups	20	0	6	0
Onion	1 cup	54	2	12	0
Mushrooms	1 cup ckd	42	3.4	8	0.8
Salsa	4 tbsp	16	0	4	0
Spinach	1 cup ckd	42	5.4	6.8	0.4
Peas	1/2 cup	57	4	10	0
Tomato	1 med	24	1	5	0

DAIRY PRODUCTS

Food Item	Qty	Calories	Protein	Carbs	Fat
Milk, skim	1 cup	90	8	12	1
milk, 1% lowfat	1 cup	100	8	11	2
cheese, American, nonfat	2 slices	80	12	6	0
cheese, American, lowfat	1.5 slices	105	9	3	6
cottage cheese, 1% lowfat	5 oz	100	17.5	6	1.3
cottage cheese, nonfat	5 oz	100	16.2	7.5	0
cream cheese, nonfat	3 oz	90	16	6	3
sour cream, non fat	2 tbsp	20	2.5	2.5	0
Yogurt, 1% lowfat	8 oz (1)	250	9	50	2
Yogurt, nonfat	8 ox (1)	100	8	17	0
Yogurt, frozen, nonfat	1 cup	180	8	38	0

FATS

Food Item	Qty	Calories	Protein	Carbs	Fat
Olive Oil	1 tbsp	120	0	0	13.8
Canola Oil	1 tbsp	120	0	0	14
Sunflower Oil	1 tbsp	120	0	0	14
Safflower Oil	1 tbsp	120	0	0	14
Flaxseed Oil	1 tbsp	130	0	0	14
Peanuts	1/2 cup	428	17.3	15.7	36.3
Peanut Butter, natural	1 tbsp	100	3.5	3.5	8
Cashews	1/2 cup	394	10.5	22.4	31.7
Udo's essential oil blend	1 tbsp	134	0	0	14.2
Salad Dress., Italian	1 tbsp	82	0	2	9
Salad Dress., Bals vingr	1 tbsp	75	0	0.5	8
Salad Dress., light Italian	3 tbsp	12	0	3	0

REFERENCES

Nix, Staci. Williams' Basic Nutrition & Diet Therapy. St. Louis, MO: Elsevier Mosby, 2005. Print.

Campbell, Neil A., Brad Williamson, and Robin J. Heyden. Biology: Exploring Life. Needham, MA: Pearson, 2004. Print.

"Vegetables and Fruits." The Nutrition Source. N.p., n.d. Web. 13 Apr. 2016.

."Micronutrients: What They Are and Why They're Essential / Nutrition / Vitamins and Minerals." Micronutrients: What They Are and Why They're Essential / Nutrition / Vitamins and Minerals. N.p., n.d. Web. 13 Apr. 2016.

"How to Calculate How Much Water You Should Drink." Let's Talk Total Rewards. N.p., n.d. Web. 13

"Calorie Calculator - Daily Calorie Needs." Calorie Calculator. N.p., n.d. Web. 13 Apr. 2016.Apr. 2016.

"Low-Calorie Diet." WebMD. N.p., n.d. Web. 13 Apr. 2016.

"10 Things You Don't Know about Calories." Shape Magazine. N.p., 23 Apr. 2009. Web. 13 Apr. 2016.

"Fiber: How Much Do I Need?" WebMD. N.p., n.d. Web. 13 Apr. 2016.

"Chapter 7 Carbohydrates." Chapter 7 Carbohydrates. N.p., n.d. Web. 13 Apr. 2016.

"The Recommended Daily Intake of Calories, Carbs, Fat, Sodium & Protein."LIVESTRONG.COM. LIVESTRONG.COM, 28 Jan. 2015. Web. 13 Apr. 2016.

"How Much Protein Do You Need Every Day? - Harvard Health Blog."Harvard Health Blog RSS. N.p., 18 June 2015. Web. 13 Apr. 2016.

"Protein Intake – How Much Protein Should You Eat Per Day?" RSS 20. N.p., 20 Mar. 2014. Web. 13 Apr. 2016.

"Chapter 8 Sodium and Potassium." Chapter 8 Sodium and Potassium. N.p., n.d. Web. 13 Apr. 2016.

"Low Cholesterol Diet: How Much Cholesterol Can I Have Per Day?" - Cholesterol. N.p., n.d. Web. 13 Apr. 2016.

"PUFA Diet." LIVESTRONG.COM. LIVESTRONG.COM, 11 Aug. 2015. Web. 13 Apr. 2016.

"Nutrition and Healthy Eating." Fat Grams: How to Track Dietary Fat. N.p., n.d. Web. 13 Apr. 2016.

"Know Your Fats." Know Your Fats. N.p., n.d. Web. 13 Apr. 2016.

"U.S. Food and Drug Administration." Lowering Salt in Your Diet. N.p., n.d. Web. 13 Apr. 2016.

"Nutrition and Healthy Eating." Sodium: How to Tame Your Salt Habit. N.p., n.d. Web. 13 Apr. 2016.

"Cross-Reference Chart." Evaluating Research Methods in Psychology(n.d.): 158-59. Web.

NOTES

NOTES

**NOTES**

INDEX